In the Pink

By; Jackie Roppolo

"A journal of my day-to-day experience of breast cancer and chemotherapy."

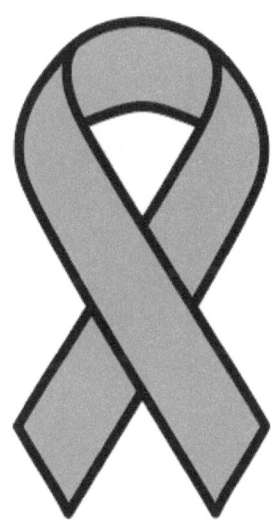

June 15 2015

I was in the shower and did a simply breast check, like I usually do and I felt a lump. "I didn't think it was there yesterday." I had my husband feel it and we both decided to quickly schedule a doctor's appointment.

They took me right in for a checkup and after taken X-rays and running tests I was told the most terrifying news that I had breast cancer. Luckily, I caught it early and it was diagnosed as stage 1 breast cancer.

*****

I decided to keep a journal of my day-to-day timeline because when I was diagnosed with breast cancer, and I tried to do some research on what to expect. I found that although there were a lot of books about breast cancer, there was nothing out there that explained or described what it felt like to not only take chemo but also to help me with what to expect going through the process each day.

Hopefully this journal help others who are diagnosed with breast cancer get, at the very least, a glimpse into what can be expected.

This is a journal of what I experienced, going through the entire 22 week process.

Disclosure

Please understand that each person is different. Please don't expect the same results and affects to happen to you. This is just my experiences of what happened to me. Hopefully this helps you with a glimpse of what to expect, going through breast cancer and its treatments.

The following entries are my own experiences with before, during and after each chemotherapy treatments

June 16, 2015

After finding out that I had breast cancer, my doctor schedule surgery for a lumpectomy and removed the lump plus a few lymph nodes to test. I was luckily told that the cancer did not spread.

My doctor suggested that I have a Smart port implanted to go through this process. Yesterday I had the safety-port surgery to implant the port just under my skin in my chest. The soreness felt as if someone punched me in the shoulder. (It's uncomfortable but manageable.

Taken a few naps but was okay to eat and drink) It was Day surgery it took about two hours but the surgery took just under an hour. Today I went back to work. my arm is still sore but I will get through the day. Thursday, I start the first cycle of chemo…Feeling very nervous.

June 17 2015

It's very early Thursday morning…Yesterday I had the safety port surgery to implant the port just under my skin in my chest. The soreness felt as if someone punched me in the shoulder. It was Day surgery it took about two hours but the surgery took just under an hour. Today I went back to work. my arm is still sore but I will get through the day. Thursday I start the first cycle of chemo. Feeling really nervous!

July 17, 2015

Today has been a very nerve-racking day I'm feeling angry and I'm scared …It just feels like a bad dream yet tomorrow I start chemotherapy. My Smart-Port is still sore in the area where they placed it but feels better today. I had a light dinner last night and a glass of wine, then had popcorn with my family and watched the women's World Cup (the US was playing)

June 17, 2015

Today is a very nerve-racking day I'm angry I'm scared ...It just feels like a bad dream yet tomorrow I start chemo.

June 18, 2015

"Chemotherapy begins today."

Today is the first day of my first chemotherapy cycle 1st of 8. The whole family is very nervous it's just an hour away from the start.

A memo from my husband

Jacquie, I know that sometimes (actually most of the time...lol), it's not easy living with me and I have to tell you that I could never live without you. You are an incredible person. You're so strong! These past few days watching you smile and laugh and enjoy being around our family, just made me realize just how strong you are...This is something that we will get through!! This is easy for you because you are SO, SO strong!!

We are here for you in every way. We love you more than anything in the world and I'm so privileged and honored to be your husband. You are strong!! You are tough!! You will get through this!!! We support you, we love you and we will be stronger from this. Baby steps! Just 7 more to go!

YOU GOT THIS!!!!!

June 18, 2015

We arrived at the office at 8:00AM. The nurses gave me anti-nausea medicine (to help with any nausea). The nurses are very friendly. My Dr. has already come in to check on me. I'm just waiting for the chemotherapy medicine to be administered. There are 9 chairs in the therapy room. 5 of the other chairs are occupied. ..at 48, I'm the youngest patient here.

About 30 minutes in… I was just given my 3rd "cocktail" before the chemo is given…

11:02am

The 1st chemo injection (red) "Adriamycin" was given. (They slowly inject it and it took about 6 minutes to inject it all). My husband sat beside me holding my hand as he began to tear up over the overwhelming life-changing process we are about to begin. …Feeling sleepy

11:28AM The second part of the chemo (Cytoxan), is now being given through intravenous. This is now a reality. So upset. Feeling sleepy from the Benadryl...taking a nap

June 19, 2015

I slept for a few hours last night. I had a headache that took a while to go away. (I took Advil and my prescriptions).

June 20, 2015

Today's agenda: I'm in for a "cocktail" From 8:00AM-2:30PM which consists of: * Injection of Nuelasta to stimulate the white blood cells to grow *Along with Dacadron and Zantac through intravenous

...Feeling pretty good this morning.

June 20, 2015

Slept through the night no headaches took the train into work today. A little dizzy right now but will eat something. I'm still drinking lots and lots of fluids (Water and Gatorade). I had to really concentrate on thinking today with my usual tasks at work... "Chemo-brain"?

June 21, 2015

I slept ok last night Feeling ok today. My bones and muscles are really sore though

June 22, 2015

Slept mostly through the night

I woke up with a slight headache and still feeling tired.
Drinking lots of fluids as I was heading to work today

At around 6:30pm "I felt like I was getting over the hump."

June 22, 2015

I was trying to stay ahead of a headache a earlier at work.

I'm feeling really good now. I feel like I got over the hump for
this 1st cycle

June 23, 2015

Still feeling good...just really tired

June 24, 2015

Still feeling good just tired I go in today to get blood work done to check my white blood cell count and probably get a boost of antibiotics to stay ahead of any potential germs.

June 24, 2015

White blood cell count low (at 1,500 should be 4-5,000) as expected...coming in tomorrow and Friday for hydration again.

June 25, 2015

8:00AM- 11:00AM

At Dr.'s office...I'm getting ready for hydration today. (2 packs of 0.9% Sodium Chloride injection USP...a 500ml pack and a 250ml pack) Just put the needle in the port still painful but wasn't as bad this time. I feel good today just a bit tired.

I started to take antibiotics last night (Cipro). She wants me to take it twice a day for 3 days.

Had blood taken again to see where my white blood cell count was today (1.16)

My Dr believes that with the Cipro, it should not go much lower... We will come back in the morning to check it again.

June 26, 2015

Feeling good... At Dr.'s for hydration again today (White Blood count is up 2.45)

June 27, 2015

I went to work today. Feeling pretty good. Just a little tired.

June 28, 2015

Feeling good again today, just a little tired.

June 29, 2015

I'm feeling good again today. I noticed a little bit more hair in my brush today.

Getting ready for work today and preparing myself mentally for Thursday's next cycle of chemo.

July 1, 2015

Last night and this morning I noticed considerable clumps of hair fallen out. I was also feeling queasy last night and this morning.

…Off to work today.

July 2 2015

Feeling a little tired from work yesterday Second round of chemo today Hair is still falling out not as bad today so far.

July 2, 2015

"Chemo Day"

8:00AM – 3:00PM Just finished cycle two of my chemotherapy treatment.

July 3, 2015

13

Was a little nauseous last night...has ginger ale and crackers...took a nausea pill...Heading in to get hydrated this morning.

I'm feeling pretty good this morning

8:00AM-1230PM today...I also had a shot to help with my white blood cell count...feeling good.

July 4 2015

It's the 4th of July and we just went to buy a temporary wig until my really good one comes in.

More hair falling out this morning (it's coming out in layers).

My bones are achy today after having that shot yesterday to help with my white blood cell count.

I feel that I'm feeling better than last week.

My family has been so supportive!

Later in the afternoon

Hair is really falling out today in clumps. My wig is coming in Tuesday, but I'm heading to a local wig shop now because not sure how much hair will fall out between now and Tuesday

July 5 2015

More hair loss today...top of head is aches. (Feels like someone is pulling my hair out)

...Other than that, I feel good, just a little tired.

July 6 2015

I'm feeling good today but my hair is really thinning...

Heading in to work today wearing a wig

...Feeling nervous

July 7 2015

I'm still feeling but good losing a lot of my hair now.

I have this bump on my forearm that feels like a blood clot (I had this just after my surgery for the port).

I will have the doctor look at it today heading in at 8:00AM.

July 8 2015

Feeling good!

I can't believe that I'm heading for a job interview now.

I got my new wig last night wearing it today, looks really life-like!

I'm going in for my two days of hydration tomorrow and Friday.

July 8 2015 (evening)

My arm started clotting.

Went to my Dr. and she wanted me get ultra sound on my arm.

Just found out It's a blood clot and I'm staying overnight at the hospital to make sure the blood clot doesn't spread.

July 9 2015

I'm still in hospital for blood clot on my arm.

My white blood cell count is at .6 (600)

...The hospital wants to keep me until Saturday on heavy doses of antibiotics and blood thinners.

...Uggh!

July 10 2015

I'm still in hospital. I'm being told until tomorrow.

Getting antibiotics and blood thinners for my blood clot.

My white blood cell count is up to 1.0 (1,000).

July 12, 2015

Finally home!

Feeling good today, just relaxing with the family.

17

July 14, 2015

I'm feeling good for the past 2 days.

…I'm just tired.

July 16 2015

I'm getting ready for my 3rd cycle of chemo today.

Feeling depressed, wish this was over.

5 more to go!!

July 16 2015

3 hours in… I had the fluids and Benadryl…etc. Now getting the round of chemo.

July 18, 2015

Had chemo and hydration Thursday and yesterday...Felt a little nauseous last night in bed.

I'm feeling better today. I have diarrhea today which I haven't had since this started and I started my period. My period is heavier; due to the blood thinner shots I'm taken.

Going to go to my daughter's soccer game and then to the New England Revolution soccer game tonight

July 19, 2015

...Still feeling good, just tired

July 21, 2015

Feeling extra tired today...went in to get hydrated...Getting fluids and starting me on antibiotics today in my IV.

I will go back in tomorrow and Thursday for same.

I'm a little anemic due to my period and blood thinner but other blood counts are ok... (Probably my last period I will ever have).

July 22, 2015

In for more hydration super nausea today they are going to give me something.

July 23, 2015

My arm started to get red again where the blood clot is. I will ask my Dr. when I'm getting hydrated today.

July 24 2015

My white blood cell count was .6 (600) yesterday so they wanted me to come back in today for antibiotics and hydration.

...Feeling much better today.

Heading back in to get antibiotics and hydration again today.

...I just can't wait for all of this to be over.

July 26, 2015

Feeling better in the past 2 days …I'm not as tired.

The blood clots are still in my arm. They seem to be a little smaller though.

July 28, 2015

I'm still feeling pretty good.

Getting ready for my last dose of the "strongest" chemo on Thursday.

…I can't wait to have this over with!

July 30, 2015

Last day of the strongest chemo cycle today. Then 4 more cycles of, the "lighter" chemo.

21

…My stomach feels funky, like it's "all tied up in knots."

July 31, 2015

Had the last round of the really strong chemo...stomach feels a little funny.

Hydration day: Going back in for hydration and my shot today.

…Then back to work!

August 1 2015

I was feeling a little nausea last night. Stomach was upset but now it's better.

August 2 2015

Really feeling tired the past couple of days. This round is really kicking my ass (in terms of being tired)...getting through it with family. So glad that was my last of the strongest chemo.

4 more rounds of the "lighter" chemotherapy to go!

I was told that my hair should start to grow back in...YAY!

Aug 4 2015

Feeling good, but still tired.

I haven't been sleeping well at all.

I can't wait for all of this to be over with!

Aug 13, 2015

Chemo day today.

Getting just the lighter chemo (but it's a new chemo for me it's called "Taxol").

I also had to take a prescription called " " (it's a sort of steroid)....5 pills last night at 9:00pm then 5 more at 3:00am and then I will take 1 more pill at 9:00pm tonight, after the chemo session today.

Aug 14 2015

Have to go to work today. (After interviewing in a wig, I got my new job).

Feeling really good today!

Just a little bit tired but I feel more like myself.

The lighter chemo I'm now taking is much easier on me.

Aug 15 2015

Off to work again today.

I'm feeling a little tired but good...day off tomorrow.

Aug 17 2015

For the past 2 days...My knees, legs and abs have been having cramps and pain that last for hours!!

I am supposed to get on a Glutamine regime which I will start tomorrow.

Note:

**Glutamine did help **

Sept 9 2015

two more chemotherapy cycles to go!

...I had a little more hair fall out today.

Sept 17 2015

25

Doing well just tired.

More hair fell out ("or, what's left of it") So I trimmed away the remaining pieces.

So overwhelming...can't wait to be finished with all of this!

Sept 24 2015

Last day of chemo!!! Yay!!!

My blood count was low today (2.5 or 2,500).

Getting extra fluids today, then coming back tomorrow for my Nuelasta shot and more fluids.

Oct 27 2015

I'm finally feeling really good.

My hair is starting to "sprout" again on my head…

I start radiation therapy on Thursday (for 6 weeks and 5 days a week).

Oct 30, 2015

2nd day of radiation...It takes about 20 minutes from parking to the treatment, to getting back in the car. (Yesterday they tattooed a few dots in the area so that they could line up the radiation beams going forward). The remaining radiation treatments went well no real side effects from the radiation. It's a simple, quick procedure, as you're in and out each day within 30 minutes or so.

...Back to work...

Over the course of days and weeks, the remaining radiation treatments went well and my aches and pains gradually got better. As my hair started to grow I had a short haircut almost like a buzz cut and then gradually to a short style haircut that I "sported" publicly. I eventually told my co-workers what I went through.

My wig was so life-like that no-one suspected I went through this ordeal, until I told them. (Although I'm sure they wondered).

(The wig was a gift from my daughter Ryann).

Oct 25, 2017

My hair has finally grown out to the length it was prior to this ordeal.

I was able to get my hair styled the way I used to have it. My hair dresser and I both cried at this ordeal and how beautiful my hair came back in.

…It's been a long journey. But I am stronger from it!

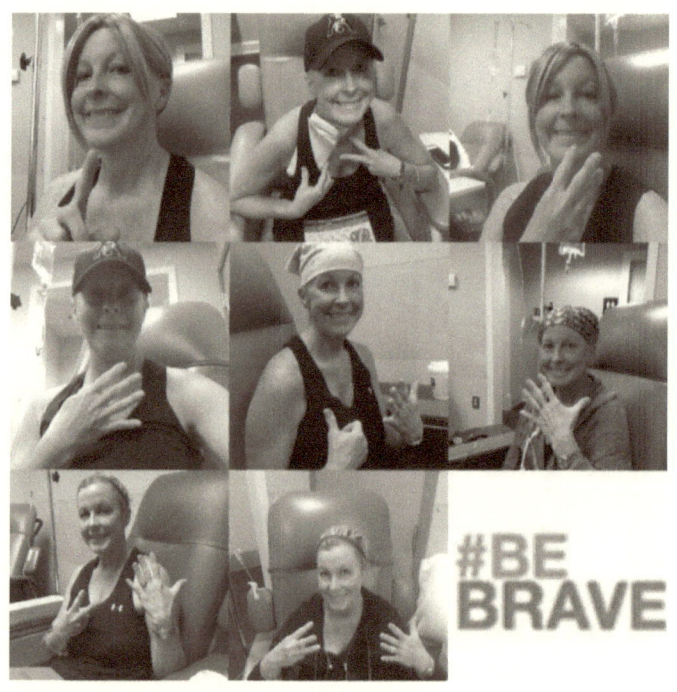

#BE
BRAVE

This 22 week journey I experienced has taught me a lot. Although I was already a very strong person and proved to me that I can get through anything!! *"Even a job interview while wearing a wig after my first round of chemo, Geez, the thought that I was able to do that now, is just amazing to me."*

Although this timeline of my journey is a raw and unedited version of my day-to-day accounts, I hope that this journal helps you like it has helped me. I am happy with the knowledge I gained, the love of my family and the satisfaction of me being able to pass this on to other strong-minded women.

I hope that this journal helps you get through this process. Be courageous! Be proud of who you are! Have a great support team of family and friends behind you.

You will get through this!

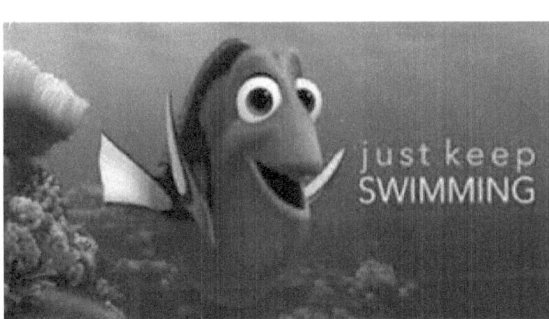

Notes:

** Neulasta: if your insurance covers it or you can afford it, take it, as it works wonders the day after chemotherapy treatments.

Special Thank you to my family: my husband Al, daughters, Bella, Ryann, her boyfriend Ben and my son Stefan.

Thank you to Dr. Dillon and The Norfolk Cancer Center for all you did to help me get through this part of my life.

Thank you to my hairdresser Stacey, from The Cuttery Hair Salon, for helping me with my hair creations.

*****A portion of the proceeds of this journal will go towards helping find a cure for breast cancer*****

www.ingramcontent.com/pod-product-compliance
Lightning Source LLC
Chambersburg PA
CBHW031335290526
45784CB00014B/2762